THE

Skinny

JUICE DIET

RECIPE BOOK

5lbs, 5 Days.
The Ultimate Kick-Start
Diet and Detox Plan to
Lose Weight & Feel Great!

The Skinny Juice Diet Recipe Book: 5lbs, 5 Days. The Ultimate Kick-Start Diet and Detox Plan to Lose Weight & Feel Great!

Copyright
Copyright © Bell & Mackenzie Publishing 2013

Disclaimer
The information and advice in this book is intended as a guide only. Any individual should independently seek the advice of a health professional before embarking on a diet.

ISBN 978-1-909855-16-8

A CIP catalogue record of this book is available from the British Library

Disclaimer
The information and advice in this book is intended as a guide only. Any individual should independently seek the advice of a doctor or health professional before embarking on any diet, detox or weight loss plan. We do not recommend a juicing plan if you are pregnant, breastfeeding or under 18 years of age. If you have an existing ailment or illness that requires medication you must first consult your doctor. Some recipes may contain nuts or traces of nuts. Those suffering from any allergies associated with nuts should avoid any recipes containing nuts or nut based oils.

Contents

Contents

Contents

Contents

Juicing

 Do you want to activate a weight loss plan that could see you lose 5lbs in just 5 days?

 Are you ready to detox your body, cleanse your digestive system and revitalise yourself both mentally and physically?

 Do you want to help alleviate the symptoms of an ailment without relying wholly on prescribed medicine?

 Do you want a fun and interesting way of increasing your essential five-a-day fruit and veg intake?

 Do you want to adopt permanent healthy eating habits that will last you a lifetime?

 Do you want to start feeling *GREAT?*

If the answer to just one of these questions is YES, then juicing could be for you.

Less of a diet and more of a way of life! Juicing is becoming increasing popular around the world and it comes with major health benefits. It's fun, it's different, it's delicious, it's easy and most importantly it works!

The Skinny Juice Diet Recipe Book will help you revitalise yourself in just 5 days with a special 5 day plan. Your body will feel rejuvenated, you could lose 5lbs in 5 days and you'll be taking the first steps to a lifelong healthy relationship with fruit and vegetables in a way you had never thought possible. This book isn't just a quick-fix diet that ends in 5 days, it contains 70 juice and smoothie recipes to kick-start a better lifestyle and introduce juicing into your existing diet.

Why Juice? – The Health Benefits

There has never been a better time to juice your way to a better life. Our media is filled with reports of the growing obesity epidemic in the western world which in turn is linked to a growing list of debilitating diseases and ailments including diabetes, high blood pressure, heart disease, high cholesterol, infertility, skin conditions and more. The super-fast pace of modern life has a lasting effect on our health with more and more of us feeling fatigued and lethargic, worsened by daily consumption of unhealthy foods. Let's face it, most of us do not consume our recommended 5 a day fruit and vegetable intake...if we did we would surely feel the benefits.

Juicing is an incredibly fast and efficient way of giving our bodies the goodness they need. Not just satisfying cravings with processed, sugar-heavy, fat-laden fast food, but instead providing vitamins, minerals and the rich nutrients which our bodies were designed to consume to help it run efficiently. By extracting these juices from fruit and vegetables our digestive systems can rapidly absorb their 100% goodness and start building and repairing our bodies fast! By stripping our diet of unhealthy processed foods weight loss becomes effortless and within days you'll feel brighter, stronger, more energetic and focussed.

At first you may be concerned about replacing your current diet with only fruit and vegetables. You do not need to worry. All our recipes are packed full of goodness and essential minerals, vitamins and nutrients that your body needs to run efficiently. The purpose of this book is not to encourage a long term vegetarian or vegan lifestyle but instead to promote the incredible health benefits of fruit and veg when their juices are extracted. There is an abundance of goodness in fruit and vegetables – we all know this, but what is so great about juicing is that we can take this goodness and harvest it in the fastest way possible – within minutes and with no cooking. Juicing really is the ultimate fast food.

Why Just 5 Days?

The Skinny Juice Diet Recipe Book provides a simple introduction to juicing (although there are also many recipes to stimulate anyone who has been juicing for some time).

A first time juicer needs a little help, guidance and motivation to get them started. Preparation is key and there can be some minor side effects you should be aware of (see *How To Get Started - Preparation*).

For most people, embarking on any kind of diet or detox plan and the prospect of committing to prolonged periods of alternative ways of eating (or in our case juicing) can be daunting and many people often give up at the first hurdle. That's not the case with this plan: The 5 Day Skinny Juice Diet Plan is short, dynamic, packed with every nutrient your body needs and is easy to follow.

It is designed as an introduction to the amazing health benefits of juicing which will deliver amazing results allowing you to potentially lose up to 5lbs in excess weight in just 5 days. Plus you will also feel incredible improvements to your general wellbeing.When the 5 days are over, the idea is you will be able to confidently incorporate juicing into your normal lifestyle every day.

The Skinny Juice Diet Recipe Book contains two parts....

Part 1 outlines the health benefits of juicing, help with sourcing the best products and tips for juicing, advice on the which type of juicer suits you best and a helpful 5 day planner to detox your body in less than a week and kick start your weight loss.

Part 2 contains over 50 additional delicious juices and smoothies which you can use in the weeks and months ahead as you continue your juicing journey and adopt juicing into your daily diet. We strongly recommend that you use the recipes in this book to supplement your normal diet as a way of life. The 5 Day Planner is a 5 day weight loss and detox plan to kick start your juicing life. It is not designed to be used for prolonged periods but as a great way to help you lose weight fast and begin adopting juicing as a long-term way of life.

How To Get Started – preparation

Preparation for the 5 day plan is essential. You are about to drastically alter the way your digestive system consumes food and your body will react accordingly. You should be prepared for some possible side effects including headaches, stomach upsets and fatigue. Not everyone experiences side effects and if you do they are normally mild and last only a few days. The good news is you can reduce the symptoms before you start the plan by following these guidelines.

• Mentally prepare yourself. If you have a positive state of mind then you are far more likely to succeed and enjoy your juicing journey. Read through all of this book including the additional recipes in the second part so you know what to expect and the type of ingredients used in the recipes.

• Where possible choose a 5 day period that is relatively quiet and not packed full of engagements that may distract you. If you attend business lunches/dinners try to schedule these so they don't conflict with your 5 day plan.

• Think and plan how you are going to make your juices. If you are at home most of the day you may be able to make each juice freshly for each stage of the plan. If however you work, then you will need to think how and when you will prepare your daytime juices. This may require you to get up earlier in the morning and prepare your drinks for the day ahead. Also you should plan where to store your drinks. You will need access to a refrigerator or a flask to keep your juices cold and

fresh.
• Tell your friends and family that you are starting the 5 day juicing plan and ask for their support.

• It is important to ease your body into the detox aspect of the 5 day plan. One week before you start the 5 day plan you should cut down on the items listed below. These should ideally be completely eliminated two days before your 5 day diet begins.

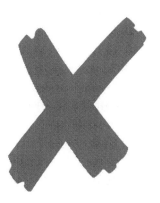

Red meat
Processed food
Dairy products
Bread
Pasta
Caffeine
Nicotine
Alcohol
Sugar
Salt

Do not be tempted to go 'cold turkey' by suddenly switching from your regular diet to the 5 day juicing plan. One week before you start you should increase your consumption of raw fruit and vegetables, particularly leafy green veg. Vegetable soups are an ideal way of increasing vegetable intake. Start drinking lots more water. As part of your 5 juice plan you will be required to drink multiple glasses of water.

Decide where you are going to buy your produce. The best sourced fruit and veg and most likely cheapest will be from your local farmers market. Research where the nearest one is to you and which day of the week it runs so you can prepare your 5 day plan accordingly. Remember you may not be able to source every ingredient so take note of any substitutes. If you are buying your produce from a supermarket/grocery store then thoroughly investigate their fruit and vegetable areas. It may be that they are stocked with fresher produce at a particular time of day. Try to source organic produce if you can afford to.

Ease back into your regular diet. It is equally important after the 5 day plan that you gently adjust your body back into digesting solid foods. The same guidelines above apply after completing the plan. So start off with light meals, predominantly raw fruit and veg, continue to drink plenty of water and slowly introduce heavier foods such as dairy, pasta and meat. We hope you will continue to incorporate juice into your daily diet. We recommend a juice a day so starting this ritual immediately after the 5 day plan will set you on the road to juicing for life. In the second part of this book are a further 50+ recipes to accompany you on your juicing journey.

Which Juicer/Blender?

There are currently three main types of juicer on the market today.

- **Centrifugal Juicer**
- **Masticating Juicer**
- **Twin Gear Juicer**

Centrifugal Juicer

Works by pressing fruit and vegetables down through a central feeder to a blade which runs at high speeds to cut the fruit and veg and displaces the pulp. These are generally the most popular type of juicers because they are very fast and fairly easy to clean. The speed at which they cut the fruit and veg however, creates a higher temperature and air which in turn reduces the length of time that you can preserve your juice. Centrifugal juicers can process most whole fruits and vegetables but can be noisy due to the powerful motor. These appliances are not suitable for juicing wheatgrass.

Masticating Juicer
Works by grinding and crushing fruit and veg. These juicers run at much slower speeds which reduces the oxidation process (this is the chemical reaction that is started when processing your juice. The more oxidation, the less time you can keep your juice fresh) and therefore allows you to preserve your juice for longer. The feeder on these machines are smaller than on a centrifugal juicer so juicing takes a little longer, however the quality of the juice is better.

Twin Gear Juicer
Works by grinding produce between two rollers. Twin gear juicers are generally the best type of juicer you can buy but are at the higher end of the price scale. They produce good quality juice with low oxidation and are of a high build quality. Twin gear juicers are best suited to anyone who is serious about juice long-term.

Juicers can start from as little as £35/$40 up to hundreds of pounds/dollars so you should think carefully about which juicer best suits your needs before buying. It pays not to compromise on quality as frequent use of a juicer running a motor at high speeds requires a certain build quality for it to work efficiently and remain trouble free. Make sure you thoroughly research your products and read customer reviews before purchasing.

Consider the following when making your choice of juicer:

• What is your budget?
• Do you want superfast juicing or do you have more time to spend preparing?
• Are you likely to want to preserve your juice for longer periods in the fridge?
• Is the juicer easy to clean? Can the parts be placed in a dishwasher?
• Is the juicer easy to operate?

- What kind of fruit and vegetables will you be juicing and therefore can they be used efficiently in the juicer you select?
- What kind of guarantee comes with the appliance?

Blender

In case you are wondering, the job of a juicer is not to blend and vice versa the purpose of a blender is not to juice. You can juice using a blender but all produce has to be sieved through a gauze cotton cloth and the process can be time consuming, messy and produces lower quality juice.

When you are making smoothies you will also require a blender. The good news is you do not need to rush out and buy a new blender. Chances are you will have one already in your kitchen. The primary use of the blender in our smoothie recipes is to crush ice and blend other ingredients into a thicker consistency to combine with your juice. If however you do need to buy a blender we recommend good quality blenders with strong blades.

Drink Lots Of Water!

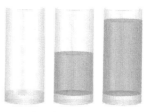

It's very important when following our 5 day planner that you drink as much water throughout the day as you can. When juicing, and especially on a juice detox/weight loss plan, your body will dispel toxins and waste (that's what we want) and so it is very important to help flush these unwanted toxins out.

We recommend consuming at least 10 glasses of water each day of the 5 day plan inbetween your daily juices. Drinking water will also help alleviate some of the side affects you may encounter when juicing on the 5 day plan.

Possible Side Effects

When you dramatically alter your diet there can be some minor side effects as your body adjusts. When juicing, most people do not experience any side effects at all. If you do experience side effects they are likely to be very mild side, but you should be aware of the following possible symptoms:

Please note: You should always consult your doctor or health professional before embarking on any diet, detox or weight loss plan. We do not recommend a juicing plan if you are pregnant, breastfeeding or under 18 years of age. If you have an existing ailment or illness that requires medication you must first consult your doctor.

Headaches
Headaches are a common side effect of juicing caused by a drop in sugar levels and lack of caffeine. Drink plenty of water.

Drop In Energy Levels
Some people when embarking on a juicing plan can feel their energy levels drop and experience periods of being tired and lethargic. This is because your body is not consuming solid food and fibre. As a result blood pressure can drop and metabolism slows down a little. This is not something you should be overly concerned about as you are only embarking on a short 5 day juicing plan. Many people actually experience the opposite and feel increased levels of energy. By the end of the 5 day plan you will reap the health benefits, so don't be disheartened.

Stomach Upset
As your body adjusts to the radical change in diet, you may experience some digestive issues including mild diarrhoea or constipation. The reduced levels of fibre are the cause of this. There should however be enough soluble fibre in our 5 day plan juices. Drinking as much water through the day as you can (minimum 10 glasses) will help with any digestive issues.

Most stomach upsets are mild and clear up very quickly.

Fibre & Protein

There is a great deal of debate about the levels of fibre and protein which are needed when embarking on a juicing diet.

Fibre

Fibre is derived from plants and helps move food through our digestive system and bowels. One of the main criticisms of a juicing plan is the lack of fibre, which can result in digestive side effects. As we are only advocating a 5 day juicing plan in this book there is no concern of any long terms side effects as a result of reduced fibre intake. Your body will get increased levels of fibre as you return to a more solid diet (incorporating regular juicing we hope).

Juice does contain fibre. There are two types of fibre – insoluble and soluble. The insoluble fibre comes from the pulp and is what helps produce regular bowel movements. The soluble fibre contained within the juices will move through your intestines and colon effectively. If you are considering a juicing diet for significantly longer than 5 days, we recommend you discuss with a health professional and research other options to increase your fibre intake. Supplements to help with this include flax seeds and chia seeds.

Protein

Protein is made up of amino acids and is essential for repair and maintenance of the body and vital for healthy skin, muscles and organs. Protein sources include, meat, milk, fish, eggs, dark green leafy vegetables, wholegrains, nuts, seeds, beans, lentils and legumes.

Our 5 day plan includes juices with protein rich produce such as broccoli, kale, spinach and celery.
Although a deficiency in protein is highly unlikely during a 5

day juice plan, you can if you prefer add protein supplements such as chia seeds and spirulina. You can source both from your local health food store.

Supplements

It is not necessary to include any additional supplements to our 5 day juicing programme. The purpose of the 5 day plan is to cleanse and detox your body and kick start weight loss over a short period of time.

However if you choose, you can supplement your 5 day juice plan with one or more of the following:

Wheatgrass – a nutrient rich grass derived from wheat. It is a good source of iron, calcium, magnesium, amino acids, chlorophyll, and vitamins A, C and E. For ease, use the powdered variety.

Spirulina – a natural algae rich in vegetable proteins and minerals. Powdered spirulina can be found in all health food stores.

Flax Seeds – good source of fibre and omega 3 fatty acids.

Chia Seeds – good source of protein, fibre and omega 3 fatty acids.

Tips

Juicing is great fun! Selecting all your favourite produce from your local farmer's market or grocery store is all part of the enjoyment. Watching your juicing appliance make quick work of all the ingredients and create the most amazing colours is magical...and that's before you have even tasted

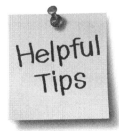

your delicious juice! There are some tips and tricks however which will make your whole juicing experience that bit easier.

• Choose the right juicer for your lifestyle and budget (see above).

• Prepare your shopping list. Take some time to select which juices you want to prepare in advance. As with all food shopping make a note of all the ingredients and quantities you need. Depending on the ingredients it's best not to shop to far in advance to ensure you are getting the freshest produce available. We recommend buying organic produce whenever you can if your budget allows. Organic produce can give a better yield and flavour of juice. Remember almost all fruit is fine to freeze too.
• Use our special 'Shopping List' for the 5 Day Skinny Juice Diet Planner. This is the simplest way to select your juices and ingredients for the next 5 days.

• If your juicer has a pulp basket, line it with a bag before juicing. This makes cleaning so much easier.

• Wash your fruit and veg before juicing. This needn't take up much time but all produce should be washed clean of any traces of bacteria, pesticides and insects.

• Prepare produce the night before for early morning juices. To save time, wash and prepare your produce the night before.

• Cut up any produce that may not fit in your juicer feeder, but only do this just before juicing to keep it as fresh as possible.

• Leave rind or peel on the fruit unless stated in the recipe (unless you find it too bitter). Check your juicer can handle rind and peel.

• Remember to use the settings on your juicer. Generally hard fruit and veg need the high speed and softer ingredients the low speed.

• Wash your juicer parts immediately after juicing. As tempting as it may be to leave it till a little later you'll be glad you took the few minutes to rinse and wash before the discarded pulp and peel has hardened.

• Substitute where you need to. If you can't source a particular ingredient, try another instead. More often than not you will find the use of a different fruit or veg makes a really interesting and delicious alternative. In our recipes we offer some advice on alternatives but have the confidence to make your own too!

• Drink your juices slowly. This will allow your body to better absorb the nutrients.

• Exercise moderately. If you exercise on a regular basis we recommend only light exercise while embarking on the 5 day plan.

• Refrain from caffeine, alcohol, nicotine, sugar, salt and non-prescribed medicines.

• Some juices are sweeter than others and it's a fact that some of the leafy green juices can take a little getting used to. Try drinking these with a straw, you'll find them easier to drink and enjoy.

• Drink lots of water!

The Skinny Juice Diet 5 Day Planner

This is where your 5 day weight loss & detox starts. On the following pages you will find a planner for each day setting out a schedule of juices at set times followed by full recipe instructions for each juice along with some helpful tips to keep you motivated. The beginning of each day starts with a cleansing drink of hot water with either a slice of lemon, lime or ginger. Boil the water and allow to cool sufficiently to drink. If you can, use distilled water. The last drink of each day is a herbal tea to relax you before bedtime. Use whichever herbal tea you prefer. Most supermarkets/grocery/health food stores will offer a good selection.

To make things super-simple, we've put together a shopping list with the entire ingredients you will need to juice for the whole 5 day plan.

5 Day Planner Shopping List

Juice shopping list

Fruit:

36	Apples
1	Mango
5	Lemons
2	Pears
4	Oranges
1	Lime
6	Handfuls green seedless grapes
6	Handfuls strawberries
2	Handfuls blueberries

Herbs & Salad:

3	Cucumbers
2	Baby gem lettuce
2	Handfuls fresh mint leaves
4	Handfuls watercress
2	Handfuls fresh flat leaf parsley
1	Large piece fresh ginger root (8in/20cm)

Vegetables:

27	Carrots
5	Beetroot
1	Courgette/zucchini
1	Parsnip
3	Stalks celery
24	Stalks kale
2	Handfuls spinach

Extras:

1	Box mixed herbal teas
1	Large bag of ice (if you prefer your juice poured over ice)

20

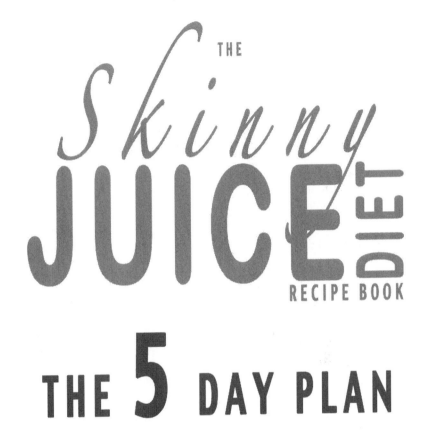

THE
Skinny
JUICE DIET
RECIPE BOOK

THE 5 DAY PLAN

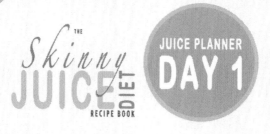

JUICE PLANNER
DAY 1

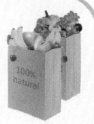

RISE & SHINE DRINK: HOT WATER WITH LEMON

8AM JUICE: EARLY RISER

MID-MORNING JUICE: GREEN MEDLEY

2PM LUNCH JUICE: GINGER BEET JUICE

5PM DINNER JUICE: CARROT FANTASTIC

EARLY EVENING JUICE: STRAWBERRY SALAD

BEDTIME DRINK: HOT HERBAL DRINK

It's day 1 of your 5 day plan. Think positive and take pleasure from preparing your first juices. Remember to drink plenty of water throughout the day.

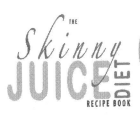
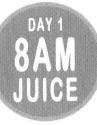
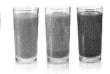

THE
Skinny
JUICE DIET
RECIPE BOOK

DAY 1
8AM
JUICE

EARLY RISER

INGREDIENTS:
2 Golden Delicious, Pink Lady or Gala apples
2 carrots
¼ lemon
½ stalk celery

DIRECTIONS:
Give the ingredients a good rinse.
Chop everything to a useable size depending on the size of your juicer.
Place into your juicer & juice.

This is a really light refreshing juice.
Great for mornings!

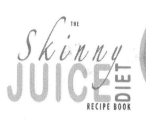 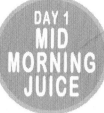 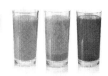

GREEN MEDLEY

INGREDIENTS:
4 stalks kale
1 handful green seedless grapes
2 Golden Delicious, Pink Lady or Gala apples
¼ cucumber

DIRECTIONS:
Give the ingredients a good rinse.
Chop everything to a useable size depending on the size of your juicer.
Place into your juicer & whizz.

Kale is packed with super nutrient qualities. It can sometimes be a little bitter so substitute with spinach if you prefer.

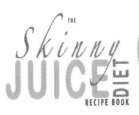 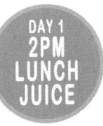 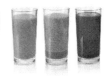

GINGER BEET JUICE

INGREDIENTS:
2 beetroots
2 carrots
1 Golden Delicious, Pink Lady or Gala apple
¼ cucumber
1 inch/2.5 cm piece fresh ginger root.

DIRECTIONS:
Give the ingredients a good rinse.
Chop everything to a useable size depending on the size of your juicer.
Place into your juicer & juice.

Ginger is an excellent detox ingredient which can reduce the risk of coughs and colds.

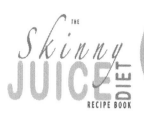  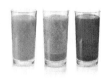

THE
Skinny
JUICE DIET
RECIPE BOOK

DAY 1
5PM
DINNER
JUICE

CARROT FANTASTIC

INGREDIENTS:
5 carrots
1 Golden Delicious, Pink Lady or Gala apple
¼ cucumber
¼ lemon

DIRECTIONS:
Give the ingredients a good rinse.
Chop everything to a useable size depending on the size of your juicer.
Place into your juicer & juice.

The protective qualities of the beta-carotenes in carrots can help reduce the risk of skin cancer.

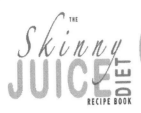

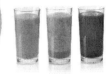

STRAWBERRY SALAD

INGREDIENTS:
1 ripe pear
¼ lemon
1 baby gem lettuce
1 small handful fresh mint leaves
1 handful ripe strawberries
1 Golden Delicious, Pink Lady or Gala apple

DIRECTIONS:
Give the ingredients a good rinse.
Chop everything to a useable size depending on the size of your juicer.
Place into your juicer & juice.

As well as being high in vitamin C, strawberries are also a good source of folate, potassium, dietary fibre, and manganese.

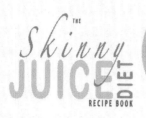

THE
Skinny
JUICE DIET
RECIPE BOOK

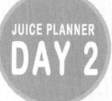

JUICE PLANNER
DAY 2

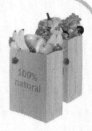

100% natural

RISE & SHINE DRINK:	HOT WATER WITH LIME
8AM JUICE:	CITRUS TWIST
MID-MORNING JUICE:	KING KALE
2PM LUNCH JUICE:	SKIN CLEANSER
5PM DINNER JUICE:	GREEN STABILISER
EARLY EVENING JUICE:	PINEAPPLE SPARK
BEDTIME DRINK:	HOT HERBAL DRINK

If the timings of our planner don't suit you, feel free to make adjustments as long as you leave 2-3 hours between juices and consume all 6 drinks in a day (plus water).

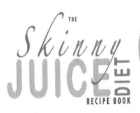
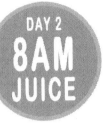

CITRUS TWIST

INGREDIENTS:
2 Golden Delicious, Pink Lady or Gala apples
1 handful green seedless grapes
¼ lemon
1 inch/2cm fresh root ginger

DIRECTIONS:
Give the ingredients a good rinse.
Chop everything to a useable size depending on the size
of your juicer.
Place into your juicer & juice.

Lemons have strong antibacterial,
antiviral, and immune-boosting powers as
well as being an aid to digestion.

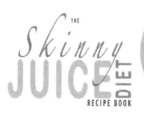 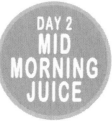 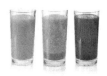

KING KALE

INGREDIENTS:
4 stalks kale
½ pineapple
1 handful watercress
1 Golden Delicious, Pink Lady or Gala apple
¼ cucumber

DIRECTIONS:
Give the ingredients a good rinse.
Chop everything to a useable size depending on the size of your juicer.
Place into your juicer & juice.

Super-food Kale is a king amongst vegetables with its intense levels of beta carotene, vitamin K, vitamin C, and calcium.

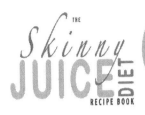

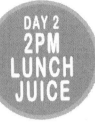
**DAY 2
2PM
LUNCH
JUICE**

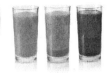

SKIN CLEANSER

INGREDIENTS:
3 carrots
2 Golden Delicious, Pink Lady or Gala apples
¼ cucumber

DIRECTIONS:
Give the ingredients a good rinse.
Chop everything to a useable size depending on the size
of your juicer.
Place into your juicer & juice.

Widely used in beauty treatments
cucumber can help to improve the quality
of the skin's complexion.

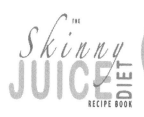 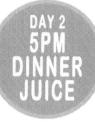 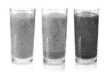

GREEN STABILISER

INGREDIENTS:
4 stalks kale
1 handful spinach
1 handful watercress
1 carrot
2 Golden Delicious, Pink Lady or Gala apples

DIRECTIONS:
Give the ingredients a good rinse.
Chop everything to a useable size depending on the size of your juicer.
Place into your juicer & juice.

This juice is packed with vitamin and mineral density which will help stablise your system.

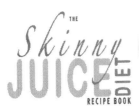
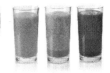
PINEAPPLE SPARK

INGREDIENTS:
½ fresh pineapple
½ celery stalk
2 oranges
¼ lemon
1 inch/2.5cm piece fresh ginger root

DIRECTIONS:
Give the ingredients a good rinse.
Peel the oranges, leave the pith on. Discard the rind.
Chop everything to a useable size depending on the size
of your juicer.
Place into your juicer & juice.

The fresh ginger in this juice sparks a
lovely flavour complement against the
sweet pineapple.

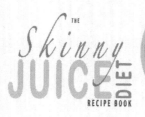

JUICE PLANNER
DAY 3

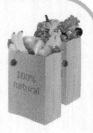

100% natural

RISE & SHINE DRINK:	**HOT WATER & GINGER SLICE**
8AM JUICE:	**EARLY RISER**
MID-MORNING JUICE:	**GOOD GREEN BEGINNINGS**
2PM LUNCH JUICE:	**GREEN MEDLEY**
5PM DINNER JUICE:	**REAL ROOTS**
EARLY EVENING JUICE:	**BERRY POWER**
BEDTIME DRINK:	**HOT HERBAL DRINK**

By the end of today you will be more than half way through the 5 day plan - well done! If you find you are suffering from any minor side effects such as stomach upset, headaches or feeling tired, remember these are normal and will pass. Keep drinking lots of water.

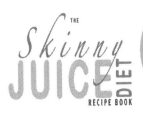 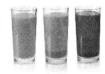

EARLY RISER

INGREDIENTS:
2 Golden Delicious, Pink Lady or Gala apples
2 carrots
¼ lemon
½ stalk celery

DIRECTIONS:
Give the ingredients a good rinse.
Chop everything to a useable size depending on the size
of your juicer.
Place into your juicer & juice.

This is a really light refreshing juice.
Great for mornings!

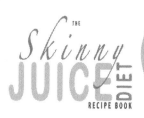 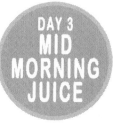 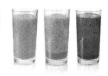

GOOD GREEN BEGINNINGS

INGREDIENTS:
¼ cucumber
½ courgette/zucchini
1 small handful fresh flat leaf parsley
¼ celery stalk
1 small handful green seedless grapes
2 Golden Delicious, Pink Lady or Gala apples
¼ lime

DIRECTIONS:
Give the ingredients a good rinse.
Peel the lime, leave the pith on. Discard the rind.
Chop everything to a useable size depending on the size of your juicer.
Place into your juicer & juice.

Parsley is the surprise package in this juice as a good source of antioxidants, folic acid & vitamin K, C & A.

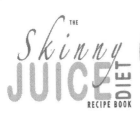
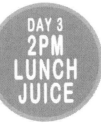
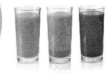
GREEN MEDLEY

INGREDIENTS:
4 stalks kale
1 handful green seedless grapes
2 Golden Delicious, Pink Lady or Gala apples
¼ cucumber

DIRECTIONS:
Give the ingredients a good rinse.
Chop everything to a useable size depending on the size of your juicer.
Place into your juicer & whizz.

Kale is packed with super nutrient qualities. It can sometimes be a little bitter so substitute with spinach if you prefer.

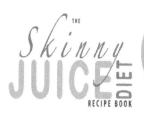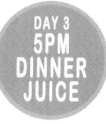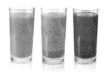

THE

Skinny
JUICE DIET
RECIPE BOOK

DAY 3
5PM
DINNER
JUICE

REAL ROOTS

INGREDIENTS:
2 Golden Delicious, Pink Lady or Gala apples
1 carrot
1 parsnip
½ beetroot

DIRECTIONS:
Give the ingredients a good rinse.
Chop everything to a useable size depending on the size of your juicer.
Place into your juicer & juice.

The vitamin rich root vegetables in this juice comprise a triple defense against ailments.

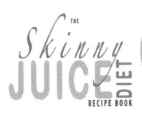

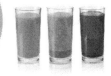

BERRY POWER

INGREDIENTS:
1 handful blueberries
2 handfuls strawberries
½ ripe mango
1 Golden Delicious, Pink Lady or Gala apple

DIRECTIONS:
Give the ingredients a good rinse.
Peel the mango, de-stone and discard the rind.
Chop everything to a useable size depending on the size of your juicer.
Place into your juicer & whizz.

As well as being delicious, there is evidence to suggest blueberries can reduce inflammation and the risk of cancer.

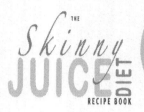
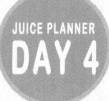
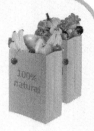

RISE & SHINE DRINK: HOT WATER & LEMON
8AM JUICE: STRAWBERRY SALAD
MID-MORNING JUICE: GINGER BEET JUICE
2PM LUNCH JUICE: GREEN STABILISER
5PM DINNER JUICE: SKIN CLEANSER
EARLY EVENING JUICE: PINEAPPLE SPARK
BEDTIME DRINK: HOT HERBAL DRINK

By now your body will have shifted many of its toxins and inpurities. If your goal is to lose weight, don't be tempted to stand on your scales until the day after the 5 day plan has ended.

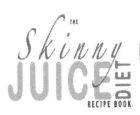 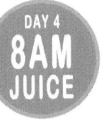 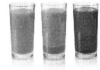
STRAWBERRY SALAD

INGREDIENTS:
1 ripe pear
¼ lemon
1 baby gem lettuce
1 small handful fresh mint leaves
1 handful ripe strawberries
1 Golden Delicious, Pink Lady or Gala apple

DIRECTIONS:
Give the ingredients a good rinse.
Chop everything to a useable size depending on the size of your juicer.
Place into your juicer & juice.

As well as being high in vitamin C, strawberries are also a good source of folate, potassium, dietary fibre, and manganese.

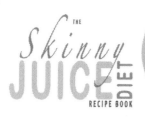 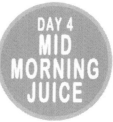 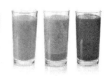

GINGER BEET JUICE

INGREDIENTS:
2 beetroots
2 carrots
1 Golden Delicious, Pink Lady or Gala apple
¼ cucumber
1 inch/2.5 cm piece fresh ginger root

DIRECTIONS:
Give the ingredients a good rinse.
Chop everything to a useable size depending on the size of your juicer.
Place into your juicer & juice.

Ginger is an excellent detox ingredient which can reduce the risk of coughs and colds.

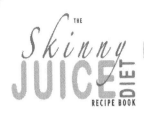 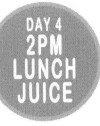 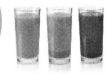

GREEN STABILISER

INGREDIENTS:
4 stalks kale
1 handful spinach
1 handful watercress
1 carrot
2 Golden Delicious, Pink Lady or Gala apples

DIRECTIONS:
Give the ingredients a good rinse.
Chop everything to a useable size depending on the size of your juicer.
Place into your juicer & juice.

This juice is packed with vitamin and mineral density which will help stablise your system.

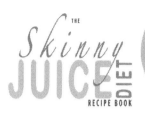 THE
Skinny
JUICE DIET
RECIPE BOOK

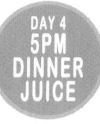
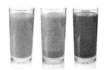

SKIN CLEANSER

INGREDIENTS:
3 carrots
2 Golden Delicious, Pink Lady or Gala apples
¼ cucumber

DIRECTIONS:
Give the ingredients a good rinse.
Chop everything to a useable size depending on the size
of your juicer.
Place into your juicer & juice.

Widely used in beauty treatments
cucumber can help to improve the quality
of the skin's complexion.

THE
Skinny
JUICE DIET
RECIPE BOOK

**DAY 4
EARLY
EVENING
JUICE**

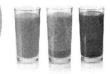

PINEAPPLE SPARK

INGREDIENTS:
½ fresh pineapple
½ celery stalk
2 oranges
¼ lemon
1 inch/2.5cm piece fresh ginger root

DIRECTIONS:
Give the ingredients a good rinse.
Peel the oranges, leave the pith on. Discard the rind.
Chop everything to a useable size depending on the size
of your juicer.
Place into your juicer & juice.

The fresh ginger in this juice sparks a
lovely flavour complement against the
sweet pineapple.

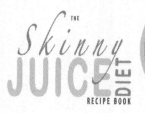

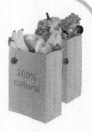

RISE & SHINE DRINK:	HOT WATER & LIME
8AM JUICE:	CITRUS TWIST
MID-MORNING JUICE:	KING KALE
2PM LUNCH JUICE:	GOOD GREEN BEGINNINGS
5PM DINNER JUICE:	CARROT FANTASTIC
EARLY EVENING JUICE:	BERRY POWER
BEDTIME DRINK:	HOT HERBAL DRINK

It's the final day of your 5 day juicing plan. Already you will be picking out which juices are your favourites. Remember there are 50 more juices and smoothies in the second part of this book.

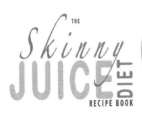
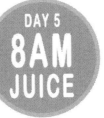

DAY 5
8AM
JUICE

CITRUS TWIST

INGREDIENTS:
2 Golden Delicious, Pink Lady or Gala apples
1 handful green seedless grapes
¼ lemon
1 inch/2cm fresh root ginger

DIRECTIONS:
Give the ingredients a good rinse.
Chop everything to a useable size depending on the size of your juicer.
Place into your juicer & juice.

Lemons have strong antibacterial, antiviral, and immune-boosting powers as well as being an aid to digestion.

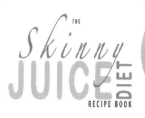 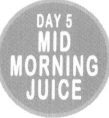 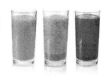

KING KALE

INGREDIENTS:
4 stalks kale
½ pineapple
1 handful watercress
1 Golden Delicious, Pink Lady or Gala apple
¼ cucumber

DIRECTIONS:
Give the ingredients a good rinse.
Chop everything to a useable size depending on the size of your juicer.
Place into your juicer & juice.

Super-food Kale is a king amongst vegetables with its intense levels of beta carotene, vitamin K, vitamin C, and calcium.

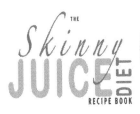

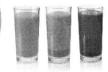

GOOD GREEN BEGINNINGS

INGREDIENTS:
¼ cucumber
½ courgette/zucchini
1 small handful fresh flat leaf parsley
¼ celery stalk
1 small handful green seedless grapes
2 Golden Delicious, Pink Lady or Gala apples
¼ lime

DIRECTIONS:
Give the ingredients a good rinse.
Peel the lime, leave the pith on. Discard the rind.
Chop everything to a useable size depending on the size
of your juicer.
Place into your juicer & juice.

Parsley is the surprise package in this juice as a good source of antioxidants, folic acid & vitamin K, C & A.

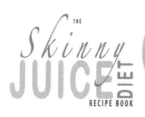 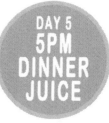 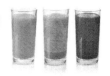

THE

Skinny

JUICE DIET

RECIPE BOOK

DAY 5
5PM
DINNER
JUICE

CARROT FANTASTIC

INGREDIENTS:
5 carrots
1 Golden Delicious, Pink Lady or Gala apple
¼ cucumber
¼ lemon

DIRECTIONS:
Give the ingredients a good rinse.
Chop everything to a useable size depending on the size of your juicer.
Place into your juicer & juice.

The protective qualities of the beta-carotenes in carrots can help reduce the risk of skin cancer.

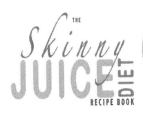

THE
Skinny
JUICE DIET
RECIPE BOOK

DAY 5
EARLY
EVENING
JUICE

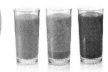

BERRY POWER

INGREDIENTS:
1 handful blueberries
2 handfuls strawberries
½ ripe mango
1 Golden Delicious, Pink Lady or Gala apple

DIRECTIONS:
Give the ingredients a good rinse.
Peel the mango, de-stone and discard the rind.
Chop everything to a useable size depending on the size of your juicer.
Place into your juicer & whizz.

As well as being delicious there is evidence to suggest blueberries can reduce inflammation and the risk of cancer.

JUICE
FOR LIFE

Juice For Life – 50+ More Juice & Smoothie Recipes To Accompany You On Your Juicing Journey

Now that you have completed the 5 day plan you should be feeling revitalised, healthy, focussed and a few pounds lighter. There are different approaches to your juicing journey from now on. Some continue to make juicing the main focus of their diet eating little in the way of the solid foods (we recommend consulting with a health professional before adopting this route), while others return to their 'normal' diet but embark on a juice fast/detox a couple of times a year. The most common route is to introduce juicing as a regular part of a daily diet. This could be starting the day with an energy boosting juice, perhaps replacing lunch with a nutrient packed green veg drink or overall reducing the intake of meat, processed food and dairy in favour of delicious, nutritious fruit and veg.

Whichever route you decide to take, we hope that the 5 day plan has given you a great introduction to the world of juicing and that you choose to juice for life and reap the health benefits.

In the following pages are 50+ more great tasting juices and smoothies that you can use beyond the 5 day plan and start you on your juicing journey. Feel free to experiment and substitute ingredients that you can better source or to suit your own taste. **Enjoy!**

Fruit Based Juices

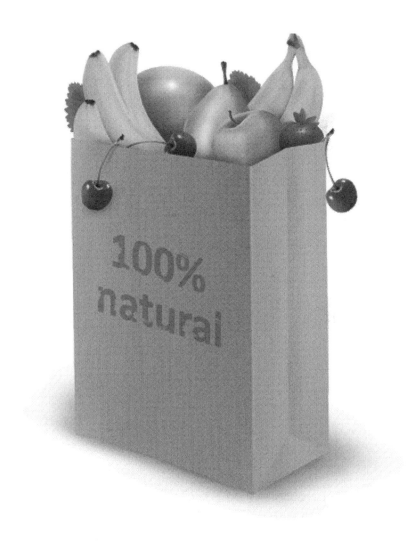

Grapefruit
Love
Serves 1

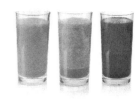

Ingredients:

2 oranges
2 yellow or ruby grapefruits
1 Golden Delicious, Pink Lady or Gala apple

Method:

• Give the ingredients a good rinse.
• Peel the oranges & grapefruits, leave the pith on. Discard the rind.
• Chop everything to a useable size depending on the size of your juicer.
• Place into your juicer & juice.

This juice is a great source of vitamin C, giving a double blast from both the oranges and grapefruits.

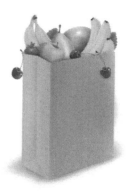

56

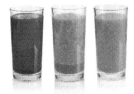

Melon & Cinnamon Swirl

Serves 1

Method:

- Give the ingredients a good rinse.
- Chop everything to a useable size depending on the size of your juicer.
- Place into your juicer & juice.

Widely used in traditional medicine, cinnamon is thought to help control blood glucose levels

Ingredients:

1 sweet potato
¼ cantaloupe melon
1 Golden Delicious, Pink Lady or Gala apple
1 ripe pear
1 inch/2.5 cm piece fresh ginger root
½ tsp ground cinnamon

Triple
Greenery
Serves 1

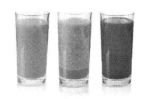

Ingredients:

¼ lime
1 small handful
fresh sage leaves
½ celery stalk
½ head crisp green
pointed cabbage
1 Golden Delicious,
Pink Lady or Gala
apple
1 ripe pear

Method:

• Give the ingredients a good rinse.
• Peel the lime, leave the pith on. Discard the rind.
• Chop everything to a useable size depending on the size of your juicer.
• Place into your juicer & juice.

This super-juice benefits from the triple green turbo charge of celery, cabbage & pear.

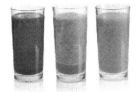

Ruby Red Juice
Serves 1

Method:

- Give the ingredients a good rinse.
- Peel the orange, leave the pith on. Discard the rind.
- Chop everything to a useable size depending on the size of your juicer.
- Place into your juicer & juice.

Fennel is believed to have medical qualities which can reduce the risk of some cancers.

Ingredients:

¼ watermelon
1 whole orange
1 Golden Delicious, Pink Lady or Gala apple
¼ fennel bulb

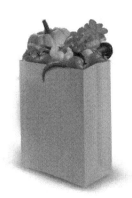

Hit Me Up
Serves 1

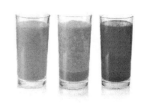

Ingredients:

1 carrot
1 Golden Delicious,
Pink Lady or Gala
apple
¼ lemon
1 baby gem lettuce
2 handfuls
strawberries

Method:

•Give the ingredients a good rinse.
•Chop everything to a useable size depending on the size of your juicer.
•Place into your juicer & juice

This juice is jam-packed with sweetness & goodness.

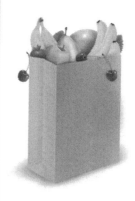

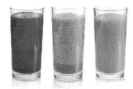

Cherry
Body
Booster
Serves 1

Method:

- Give the ingredients a good rinse.
- Chop everything to a useable size depending on the size of your juicer.
- Place into your juicer & whizz.

Ingredients:

1 Golden Delicious, Pink Lady or Gala apple
1 ripe pear
3 handfuls cherries, de-stoned

This is a really refreshing juice, which is a great body booster when your energy levels feel low.

Kiwi Power
Serves 1

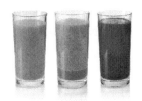

Ingredients:

**3 ripe kiwis
(remove the skin
if you prefer)
1 orange
1 Golden
Delicious, Pink
Lady or Gala apple
¼ cucumber**

Method:

• Give the ingredients a good rinse.
• Peel the orange, leave the pith on. Discard the rind.
• Chop everything to a useable size depending on the size of your juicer.
• Place into your juicer & whizz.

Kiwifruit is a rich source of vitamins C & A which, when coupled with the vitamin packed oranges, makes for an awesome power juice.

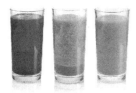

Almond
Muscle
Builder
Serves 1

Method:

- Give the ingredients a good rinse.
- Peel the orange, leave the pith on. Discard the rind.
- Drain the almonds.
- Chop everything to a useable size depending on the size of your juicer.
- Place into your juicer & juice.

Almonds are a rich source of vitamin E and are believed to have health benefits which include improved complexion.

Ingredients:

1 orange
½ sweet potato
¼ cucumber
1 Golden Delicious, Pink Lady or Gala apple
2 handfuls raw almonds (soak in water overnight)

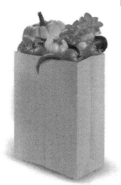

Basil Brain Booster

Serves 1

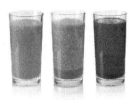

Ingredients:

¼ lemon
2 Golden Delicious,
Pink Lady or Gala
apples
½ cucumber
1 handful fresh
basil leaves

Method:

•Give the ingredients a good rinse.
•Chop everything to a useable size depending on the size of your juicer.
•Place into your juicer & juice.

Basil contains antioxidant, antiviral, and antimicrobial properties, which can help keep you healthy and boost your brain power.

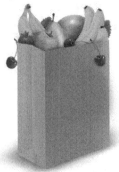

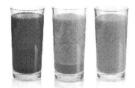

Bang Bang Juice

Serves 1

Method:

- Give the ingredients a good rinse.
- Chop everything to a useable size depending on the size of your juicer.
- Place into your juicer & juice.

Ingredients:

½ celery stalk
½ cucumber
1 Golden Delicious, Pink Lady or Gala apple
2 beetroot
¼ lemon
½ small red chilli

Adjust the chilli to suit your own taste but remember part of the joy of this juice is the natural 'high' the fresh chilli 'bang' will give you.

Love Your Liver

Serves 1

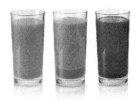

Ingredients:

1 handful
strawberries
1 large wedge
watermelon (about
an eighth)
1 Golden Delicious,
Pink Lady or Gala
apple
½ parsnip
¼ lemon

Method:

• Give the ingredients a good rinse.
• Chop everything to a useable size depending on the size of your juicer.
• Place into your juicer & juice.

This juice will get your digestion going and help cleanse your liver.

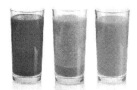

Detox Juice
Serves 1

Method:

- Give the ingredients a good rinse.
- Chop everything to a useable size depending on the size of your juicer.
- Place into your juicer & juice.

A close relation to kale, chard is another ingredient which is packed with vitamins and minerals to help detox your system.

Ingredients:

**1 handful swiss chard
1 carrot
¼ pineapple
1 Golden Delicious, Pink Lady or Gala apple
¼ cucumber**

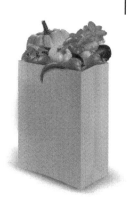

Towering
Tomatoes
Serves 1

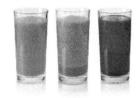

Ingredients:

3 vine ripened tomatoes
2 Golden Delicious, Pink Lady or Gala apples
½ stalk celery

Method:

• Give the ingredients a good rinse.
• Chop everything to a useable size depending on the size of your juicer.
• Place into your juicer & juice.

Tomatoes contain high levels of carotene lycopene, one of the planets most powerful natural antioxidants.

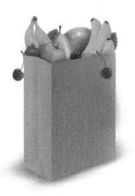

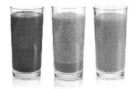

Traveling
Juice
Serves 1

Method:

- Give the ingredients a good rinse.
- Peel the oranges, leave the pith on. Discard the rind.
- Chop everything to a useable size depending on the size of your juicer.
- Place into your juicer & juice.

Ginger is used in natural remedies to help treat motion sickness.

Ingredients:

1 Golden Delicious, Pink Lady or Gala apple
2 oranges
1 garlic clove
1 inch/2cm piece ginger root

Pressure
Reliever
Serves 1

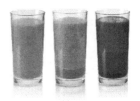

Ingredients:

**2 vine ripened
tomatoes
1 handful fresh flat
leaf parsley
2 Golden Delicious,
Pink Lady or Gala
apples
1 garlic clove**

Method:

•Give the ingredients a good
rinse.
•Chop everything to a useable
size depending on the size of
your juicer.
•Place into your juicer & juice.

*Garlic can reduce blood
pressure and cleanse the
skin. Experiment with
additional garlic if you think
you can handle it!*

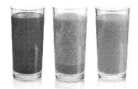

Exploding
Juice
Serves 1

Method:

- Give the ingredients a good rinse.
- Deseed the chilli and discard the seeds.
- Chop everything to a useable size depending on the size of your juicer.
- Place into your juicer & juice.

Ingredients:

1 red (bell) peppers
2 Golden Delicious, Pink Lady or Gala apples
¼ fresh pineapple
½ small red chilli

The chilli in this juice will explode in your mouth. Adjust the quantity to suit your own taste!

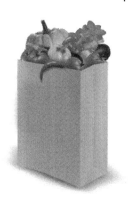

Antioxidant
Power
Juice
Serves 1

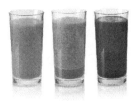

Ingredients:

5 vine ripened tomatoes
1 stalk celery
1 orange
1 Golden Delicious, Pink Lady or Gala apple
1inch/2cm piece fresh ginger root

Method:

• Give the ingredients a good rinse.
• Peel the orange, leave the pith on. Discard the peel.
• Chop everything to a useable size depending on the size of your juicer.
• Place into your juicer & juice.

Tomatoes are rich in antioxidants believed to have anti-aging qualities.

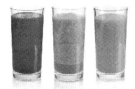

Hot
Tomatoes
Serves 1

Method:

- Give the ingredients a good rinse.
- Deseed the chilli and discard the seeds.
- Chop everything to a useable size depending on the size of your juicer.
- Place into your juicer & juice.

Adjust the chilli to suit your own taste.

Ingredients:

5 vine ripened tomatoes
½ red chilli
2 celery stalks
1 Golden Delicious, Pink Lady or Gala apple
1 carrot

Vegetable Based Juices

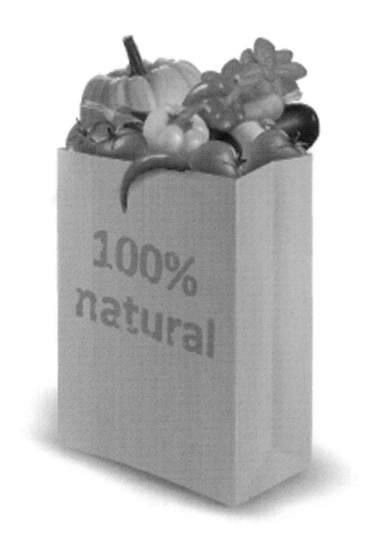

Garlic
Cleanser
Serves 1

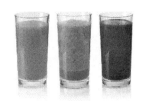

Ingredients:

1 garlic clove
3 carrots
¼ stalk celery
¼ cucumber
1 Golden Delicious,
Pink Lady or Gala
apple

Method:

•Give the ingredients a good rinse.
•Chop everything to a useable size depending on the size of your juicer.
•Place into your juicer & juice.

Garlic cleanses the skin and helps detoxify the system.

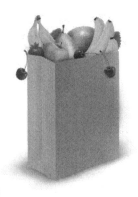

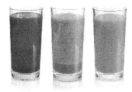

Method:

• Give the ingredients a good rinse.

• Chop everything to a useable size depending on the size of your juicer.

• Place into your juicer & juice.

The fresh basil and coriander leaves give this juice a unique blast of flavour.

Ingredients:

1 carrot
1 Golden Delicious, Pink Lady or Gala apple
½ beetroot
½ stalk celery
1 vine ripened tomato
1 handful fresh basil leaves
1 small handful fresh coriander/ cilantro leaves

Body
Booster
Serves 1

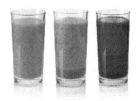

Ingredients:

½ courgette/ zucchini
1 Golden Delicious, Pink Lady or Gala apple
¼ head cauliflower
1 handful blueberries
½ orange

Method:

• Give the ingredients a good rinse.
• Peel the orange, leave the pith on. Discard the rind.
• Chop everything to a useable size depending on the size of your juicer.
• Place into your juicer & juice.

Cauliflower possesses a strong nutritional density with its high levels of dietary fibre, folate, & vitamin C.

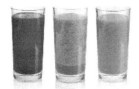

Night Vision

Serves 1

Method:

- Give the ingredients a good rinse.
- Chop everything to a useable size depending on the size of your juicer.
- Place into your juicer & juice.

Ingredients:

2 carrots
¼ cucumber
½ beetroot
¼ small red cabbage
1 Golden Delicious, Pink Lady or Gala apple

Carrots are rich in antioxidants and minerals as well as vitamin A, which according to folklore helps you see in the dark!

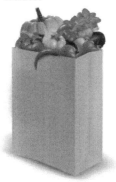

Lean &
Green
Serves 1

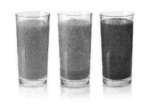

Ingredients:

3 whole kale stalks
¼ cucumber
¼ fennel bulb
1 Golden Delicious,
Pink Lady or Gala
apple
2 carrots
1 inch/2cm piece
fresh ginger

Method:

•Give the ingredients a good rinse.
•Chop everything to a useable size depending on the size of your juicer.
•Place into your juicer & juice.

The ginger gives this juice a natural 'earthy' warmth.

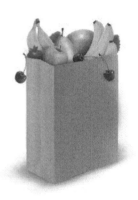

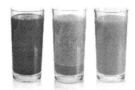

Method:

- Give the ingredients a good rinse.
- Chop everything to a useable size depending on the size of your juicer.
- Place into your juicer & juice.

Only green goodness is allowed in this super fresh juice. You could add some spinach too if you like.

Ingredients:

1 Golden Delicious, Pink Lady or Gala apple
¼ stalk celery
1 whole stalk kale
1 small handful fresh flat leaf parsley
1 ripe pear
1 baby gem lettuce

The Beet Goes On
Serves 1

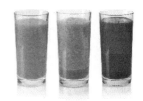

Ingredients:

2 beetroots
1 carrots
**1 Golden Delicious,
Pink Lady or Gala
apple**
½ stalk celery
**1 small handful
fresh flat leaf
parsley**

Method:

• Give the ingredients a good rinse.
• Chop everything to a useable size depending on the size of your juicer.
• Place into your juicer & juice.

The high level of antioxidants in beetroot are great for cleaning out the system.

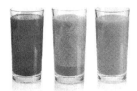

Chinese Green Juice
Serves 1

Method:

- Give the ingredients a good rinse.
- Chop everything to a useable size depending on the size of your juicer.
- Place into your juicer & juice.

Ingredients:

1 Chinese cabbage/pak choi
¼ lemon
2 Golden Delicious, Pink Lady or Gala apple

The chemical compounds that occur in pak choi are reported to help prevent skin cancer.

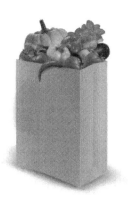

Cholesterol
Blaster
Serves 1

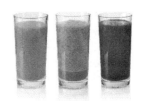

Ingredients:

**1 carrot
½ turnip
¼ cucumber
2 Golden Delicious,
Pink Lady or Gala
apples**

Method:

•Give the ingredients a good rinse.
•Chop everything to a useable size depending on the size of your juicer.
•Place into your juicer & juice.

The combined ingredients of carrot, turnip and apple will help towards lowering your cholesterol levels.

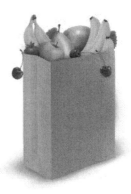

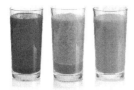

Method:

• Give the ingredients a good rinse.
• Chop everything to a useable size depending on the size of your juicer.
• Place into your juicer & juice.

Ingredients:

½ parsnip
2 carrots
1 sweet potato
½ stalk celery
1 Golden Delicious, Pink Lady or Gala apple

The natural sweetness of the parsnips & potato blend perfectly in this veggie juice.

Parsley
Pump
Serves 1

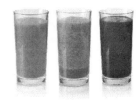

Ingredients:

1 large handful flat leaf parsley
1 carrot
¼ cucumber
2 Golden Delicious, Pink Lady or Gala apple

Method:

• Give the ingredients a good rinse.
• Chop everything to a useable size depending on the size of your juicer.
• Place into your juicer & juice.

Prized by athletes for its energy properties, parsley is extremely rich in micronutrients.

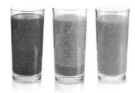

Method:

- Give the ingredients a good rinse.
- Deseed the pepper.
- Chop everything to a useable size depending on the size of your juicer.
- Place into your juicer & juice.

The cartenoids in red peppers will help improve overall skin complexion.

Ingredients:

1 red (bell) pepper
2 carrots
1 Golden Delicious, Pink Lady or Gala apple
2 spears purple sprouting or tenderstem broccoli

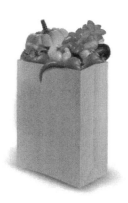

Deep
Purple
Serves 1

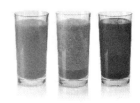

Ingredients:

**1 small aubergine/
egg plant
1 carrot
1 Golden Delicious,
Pink Lady or Gala
apple**

Method:

•Give the ingredients a good rinse.
•Chop everything to a useable size depending on the size of your juicer.
•Place into your juicer & juice.

Aubergines are packed with the antioxoidants which are believed to help prevent cancer.

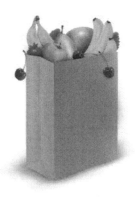

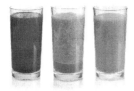

Method:

- Give the ingredients a good rinse.
- Chop everything to a useable size depending on the size of your juicer.
- Place into your juicer & juice.

Ingredients:

2 handfuls spinach
1 Golden Delicious, Pink Lady or Gala apple
2 carrots
½ beetroot

Spinach helps build muscle fibers and oxygenates the blood.

Calcium
Plus
Serves 1

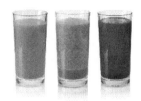

Ingredients:

6 spears purple sprouting or tenderstem broccoli
1 Golden Delicious, Pink Lady or Gala apple
1 baby gem lettuce
¼ fresh pineapple

Method:

• Give the ingredients a good rinse.
• Chop everything to a useable size depending on the size of your juicer.
• Place into your juicer & juice.

Pound for pound, broccoli contains more calcium & protein than milk.

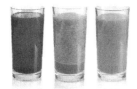

Hunger
Flash
Serves 1

Method:

- Give the ingredients a good rinse.
- Chop everything to a useable size depending on the size of your juicer.
- Place into your juicer & juice.

This is a really hearty juice which will help keep hunger at bay.

Ingredients:

¼ stalk celery
1 carrot
1 pear
1 Golden Delicious, Pink Lady or Gala apple
1 handful spinach
1 small handful fresh flat leaf parsley

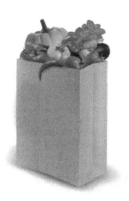

Stress
Buster
Serves 1

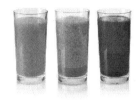

Ingredients:

**½ small green
pointed cabbage
1 carrot
2 Golden Delicious,
Pink Lady or Gala
apples**

Method:

• Give the ingredients a good rinse.
• Chop everything to a useable size depending on the size of your juicer.
• Place into your juicer & juice.

Cabbage helps to regenerate cells in the digestive system as well as healing ulcers.

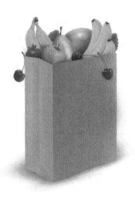

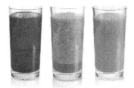

Leek & Beet Juice
Serves 1

Method:

- Give the ingredients a good rinse.
- Chop everything to a useable size depending on the size of your juicer.
- Place into your juicer & juice.

You could substitute a mild onion for the leek if you prefer.

Ingredients:

**1 leek
2 Golden Delicious, Pink Lady or Gala apples
2 beetroots**

Sweet &
Strong
Serves 1

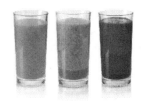

Ingredients:

½ sweet potato
1 carrot
2 radishes
½ stalk celery
1 Golden Delicious,
Pink Lady or Gala
apple
1 beetroot

Method:

• Give the ingredients a good rinse.
• Chop everything to a useable size depending on the size of your juicer.
• Place into your juicer & juice.

The sweetness comes from the sweet potato and carrots whilst the strength of this juice is in its high levels of vitamin C, potassium & betaine.

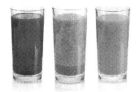

Fennel
Fantastic
Serves 1

Method:

• Give the ingredients a good rinse.

• Chop everything to a useable size depending on the size of your juicer.

• Place into your juicer & juice.

Ingredients:

½ fennel bulb
2 Golden Delicious, Pink Lady or Gala apples
1 beetroot

Fennel helps relieve the symptoms of severe headaches.

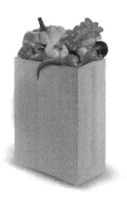

Hola Juice
Serves 1

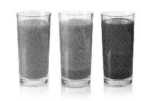

Ingredients:

¼ mild white
Spanish onion
½ beetroot
2 Golden Delicious,
Pink Lady or Gala
apples
½ stalk celery
¼ lemon

Method:

• Give the ingredients a good rinse.
• Peel the onion and discard the skin.
• Chop everything to a useable size depending on the size of your juicer.
• Place into your juicer & juice.

Say 'hola' to the Spanish onion in this juice, which contains chemicals with anti-inflammatory, anti-cholesterol and antioxidant properties.

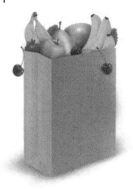

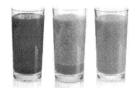

Method:

- Give the ingredients a good rinse.
- Peel the onion and discard the skin.
- Chop everything to a useable size depending on the size of your juicer.
- Place into your juicer & juice.

Studies have shown that the phenolics and flavonoids in onion may help prevent cancer.

Ingredients:

¼ mild white onion
½ sweet potato
¼ cucumber
2 carrots
1 Golden Delicious, Pink Lady or Gala apple

Greens
Unite
Serves 1

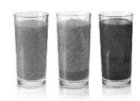

Ingredients:

**1 handful spinach
1 handful
watercress
½ green (bell)
pepper
1 carrot
¼ lemon
2 Golden Delicious,
Pink Lady or Gala
apples**

Method:

• Give the ingredients a good rinse.
• Deseed the pepper.
• Chop everything to a useable size depending on the size of your juicer.
• Place into your juicer & juice.

The chlorophyll contained in vegetable 'greens' help oxygenate the blood.

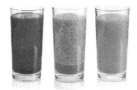

Race For
Life
Serves 1

Method:

• Give the ingredients a good rinse.
• Chop everything to a useable size depending on the size of your juicer.
• Place into your juicer & juice.

You could use yam rather than sweet potato if you like.

Ingredients:

2 radishes
½ beetroot
½ sweet potato
1 carrot
1 Golden Delicious, Pink Lady or Gala apple
½ celery stalk
¼ lemon

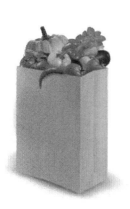

Juice
Workout
Serves 1

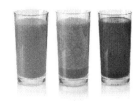

Ingredients:

½ sweet potato
2 Golden Delicious,
Pink Lady or Gala
apples
1inch/2cm slice
mild white onion
½ lemon
1inch/2cm piece
fresh root ginger

Method:

• Give the ingredients a good rinse.
• Chop everything to a useable size depending on the size of your juicer.
• Place into your juicer & juice.

This is a great juice to drink after an aerobic workout.

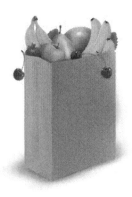

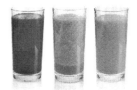

Broccoli
Feast
Serves 1

Method:

• Give the ingredients a good rinse.

• Chop everything to a useable size depending on the size of your juicer.

• Place into your juicer & juice.

Ingredients:

6 spears purple sprouting or tenderstem broccoli
1 carrot
1 Golden Delicious, Pink Lady or Gala apple
½ stalk celery

Broccoli is great for helping stave off hunger pangs.

Carrot &
Coriander
Serves 1

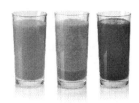

Ingredients:

**3 carrots
1 small handful
coriander/cilantro
1 handful spinach
1 handful
watercress
1 Golden Delicious,
Pink Lady or Gala
apple
1 vine ripened
tomato**

Method:

• Give the ingredients a good rinse.
• Chop everything to a useable size depending on the size of your juicer.
• Place into your juicer & juice.

Rich in fibre – carrots are great for increasing metabolism.

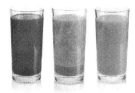

Double
Cabbage
Crusher
Serves 1

Method:

- Give the ingredients a good rinse.
- Chop everything to a useable size depending on the size of your juicer.
- Place into your juicer & juice.

Cabbages are excellent sources of vitamin K and manganese.

Ingredients:

¼ red cabbage
¼ green pointed cabbage
1 Golden Delicious, Pink Lady or Gala apple
1 beetroot
2 carrots
½ stalk celery

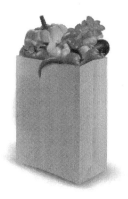

Smoothies

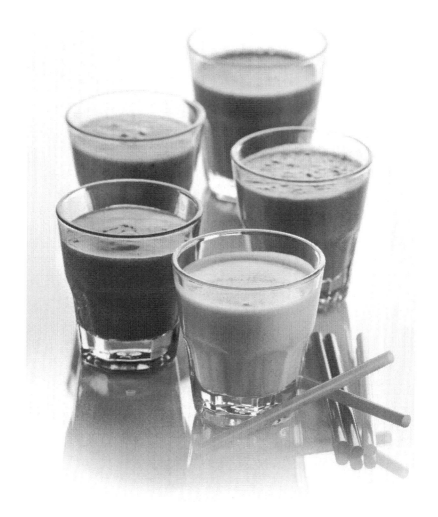

Double
Nut Energy
Smoothie
Serves 1

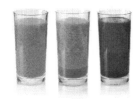

Ingredients:

3 whole stalks kale
1 Golden Delicious,
Pink Lady or Gala
apple
1 small handful
pitted dates
1 cup/250ml
natural almond
milk
½ handful raw
almonds (soaked
overnight in water)
1 tsp organic runny
honey
Handful ice cubes

Method:

• Give the ingredients a good rinse.
• Chop everything to a useable size depending on the size of your juicer.
• Put the kale and apple into your juicer & juice.
• Add the juice and all the other ingredients into a blender. Whizz until blended and smooth.

Both dates and almonds are a good source of potassium, which is an essential nutrient for all living cells.

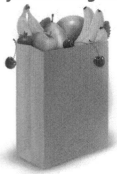

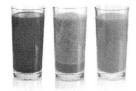

Sweet
Green
Smoothie
Serves 1

Method:

- Give the ingredients a good rinse.
- Chop everything to a useable size depending on the size of your juicer.
- Put the spinach and apple into your juicer & juice.
- Add the juice and all the other ingredients into a blender. Whizz until blended and smooth.

Manuka honey is ideal for this recipe but can be an expensive ingredient.

Ingredients:

**2 handfuls spinach
1 Golden Delicious,
Pink Lady or Gala
apple
½ banana
1 cup/250ml fat
free Greek yoghurt
1 tsp organic runny
honey
Handful ice cubes**

Raspberry & Soya Milk Smoothie

Serves 1

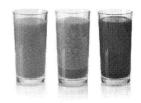

Ingredients:

2 handfuls raspberries
¼ cucumber
1 Golden Delicious, Pink Lady or Gala apple
½ banana
1 cup/250ml soya milk
Handful ice cubes

Method:

• Give the ingredients a good rinse.
• Chop everything to a useable size depending on the size of your juicer.
• Put the raspberries, cucumber and apple into your juicer & juice.
• Add the juice and all the other ingredients into a blender. Whizz until blended and smooth.

You could add kale or spinach to this smoothie if you like.

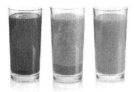

Kiwi & Blueberry Smoothie
Serves 1

Method:

- Give the ingredients a good rinse.
- Chop everything to a useable size depending on the size of your juicer.
- Put the blueberries, kiwi and apple into your juicer & juice.
- Add the juice and all the other ingredients into a blender. Whizz until blended and smooth.

Blueberries are a fantastic source of antioxidants.

Ingredients:

2 handfuls blueberries
1 kiwi (peel if you prefer)
1 Golden Delicious, Pink Lady or Gala apple
1 cup/250ml fat free Greek yoghurt
Handful ice cubes

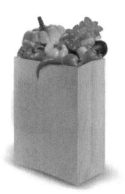

Muesli
Breakfast
Smoothie
Serves 1

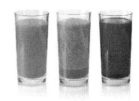

Ingredients:

**2 handfuls
blueberries
1 Golden Delicious,
Pink Lady or Gala
apple
1 cup/250ml fat
free Greek yoghurt
3 tbsp muesli
1 tsp organic runny
honey
Handful ice cubes**

Method:

• Give the ingredients a good rinse.
• Chop everything to a useable size depending on the size of your juicer.
• Put the blueberries and apple into your juicer & juice.
• Add the juice and all the other ingredients into a blender. Whizz until blended and smooth.

This breakfast smoothie will keep you going all morning.

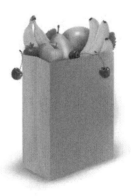

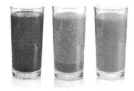

Melon & Avocado Smoothie
Serves 1

Method:

•Give the ingredients a good rinse.

•Chop everything to a useable size depending on the size of your juicer.

•Put the melon, spinach and apple into your juicer & juice.

•Add the juice and all the other ingredients into a blender. Whizz until blended and smooth.

Avocados are believed to help lower blood cholesterol levels.

Ingredients:

¼ small melon
1 Golden Delicious, Pink Lady or Gala apple
1 handful spinach
½ cup/120ml coconut water
1 avocado, peeled and stoned
Handful ice cubes

Peach &
Spinach
Smoothie
Serves 1

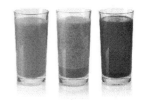

Ingredients:

1 ripe peached, de-stoned
1 handful strawberries
1 Golden Delicious, Pink Lady or Gala apple
1 handful spinach
1 cup/250ml fat free Greek yoghurt
Handful ice cubes

Method:

• Give the ingredients a good rinse.
• Chop everything to a useable size depending on the size of your juicer.
• Put the peach, strawberries, spinach and apple into your juicer & juice.
• Add the juice and all the other ingredients into a blender. Whizz until blended and smooth.

Remember you can use frozen fruit as an alternative in all your smoothie recipes.

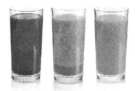

Banana & Orange Smoothie

Serves 1

Method:

- Give the ingredients a good rinse.
- Chop everything to a useable size depending on the size of your juicer.
- Peel the oranges, leave the pith on. Discard the skin.
- Put the oranges & strawberries into your juicer & juice.
- Add the juice and all the other ingredients into a blender. Whizz until smooth.

You could add a handful of spinach to your juicer for even more goodness.

Ingredients:

2 oranges, peeled
1 banana
1 handful strawberries
Handful ice cubes

Pineapple & Berry Smoothie
Serves 1

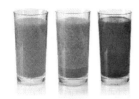

Ingredients:

½ pineapple
1 handful soft berries
1 banana
½ cup/120ml fat free Greek yoghurt
Handful ice cubes

Method:

• Give the ingredients a good rinse.
• Chop everything to a useable size depending on the size of your juicer.
• Put the pineapple & berries into your juicer & juice.
• Add the juice and all the other ingredients into a blender. Whizz until blended and smooth.

Use whichever soft berries you prefer – raspberries, strawberries or blueberries are all great.

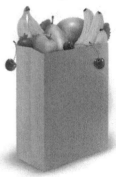

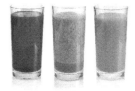

Method:

- Give the ingredients a good rinse.
- Chop everything to a useable size depending on the size of your juicer.
- Put the pineapple & blackberries into your juicer & juice.
- Add the juice and all the other ingredients into a blender. Whizz until smooth.

Feel free to use flavoured soya milk to add a different taste to your smoothie.

Ingredients:

¼ pineapple
2 handfuls blackberries
1 banana
½ cup/120ml soya milk fat yoghurt
Handful ice cubes

Lemon &
Avocado
Smoothie
Serves 1

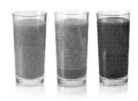

Ingredients:

**½ lemon
2 handfuls
strawberries
1 banana
½ avocado, peeled
& de-stoned
Handful ice cubes**

Method:

- Give the ingredients a good rinse.
- Chop everything to a useable size depending on the size of your juicer.
- Put the lemon & strawberries into your juicer & juice.
- Add the juice and all the other ingredients into a blender. Whizz until blended and smooth.

Double-up the lemon if you want a particularly sharp smoothie.

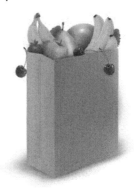

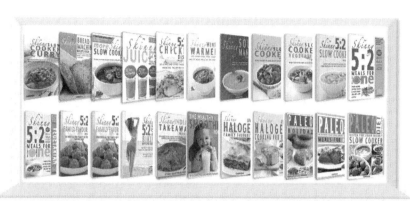

Other CookNation Titles

If you enjoyed The Skinny Juice Diet Recipe Book 5:2 we'd really appreciate your feedback. Reviews help others decide if this is the right book for them. Thank you.

You may also be interested in other titles in the CookNation series. Search 'CookNation' under Amazon.

11052584R00067

Printed in Great Britain
by Amazon.co.uk, Ltd.,
Marston Gate.